SURVIVING THE ODDS

SURVIVING THE ODDS

A True Story

Lelanie Dobson

To order additional copies of this book, contact:
Xlibris Corporation
0-800-644-6988
www.xlibrispublishing.co.uk
orders@xlibrispublishing.co.uk
300141

Contents

CHAPTER 1

Introduction

I am sitting here by myself after a long drive to visit my Dad for Christmas. My whole family from my Dad's side is here talking together, looking at their happy faces and thinking back on my life.

My name is Sarah; I was born in a small town, one year after my brother Chad. My childhood was very misguided as you can imagine. With my parents divorcing at the age of 5, we spent our Primary school days with our mother and High School day with our father. This is where my story begins.

My Mother moved to Durban after she divorced my Dad to make a new beginning for us all. My Primary days with my Mother Mandy were very entertaining. Mandy worked for a company that was involved in sports activities, which was great for me as I enjoyed my sports very much. Especially cross country, which I achieved my colors in. Mandy supported me in this and tried to attend as many events as possible.

Mandy got married a year after that she have met Jerry, to a wonderful man that accepted and loved us. We often went down the coast for holidays, until we got older. Then everything went wrong, my stepfather drank allot and was always fighting with my Mother. Every morning Mandy would say, "it is not his fault is it mine". We were all given a good life so she did not complain. He gave us a lot and also cared for us as if we were his own.

Once Chad and I finished our Primary School we moved to our Dad. He was living in Crystal Park, just outside of Benoni. Our Dad, Mitchell had a different aspect of life. He tried to teach us the right way of life. I was restricted from a lot of things as I was a girl. This is where I felt a bit of jealousy towards my brother. He was allowed to do so much more than I was. Mitchell gave me as much freedom as he saw fit, as he felt that if he lets go too much, I will go down the wrong road.

I learnt the hard way, when I decided to go out the one Friday afternoon after school with Chad to play pool at a Bar. When I returned home my Dad was already waiting for me. We had a big argument, which led to, me being sent back to my mother. I felt extremely sad as this was the only time I ever did anything wrong.

I became very rebellious and refused to listen to my mother, when I returned back to her. I only wanted my way and nobody else's way. Six months of being back with my mother, my school marks went down completely. I also started drinking and smoking

I started dating an older guy that was already out of school. My parents disapproved of him, as he had no job and was always on the beach. I avoided going to school, rather went to the beach and never studied for exams. Everything was too much for me all of a sudden. I finished grade 11, but failed. I insisted in not going back, they were very angry with me, but accepted my decision. My parents wanted to know what my plans were for the future.

It hit me so hard, when I realized what I have done. I have no experience in anything and had to make a living. So I started with waitressing to have some income.

My mother sent me away to my father for two weeks to see if I could stop thinking about my boyfriend. My father did everything possible to make me forget. He even arranged for a guy to take me out to show me what I am missing. I went back after the two weeks have passed; I then realized why I was sent to my Dad. I then decided to act maliciously towards my family and carried on dating him.

Which I in turn fell pregnant by mistake; this was not what I planned. I had to accept this first before I could confront my Mom. My mother gave me a choice to give up the baby or leave the house. This is not what I wanted to hear, especially at my age. I just left school had no income to support neither a baby nor myself. Besides I did not believe in adoption or giving up a baby, which was not asked to be here. I did not have much of a choice but to leave home. No job, no money and nowhere to go. I was scared, this was new to me. All I wanted was for my Mom to say to me, it is going to be okay—we can work though this together. But got no response from her. I was angry at that time with her.

My boyfriend then, went to his mother, she gave me not much of a choice either, it was either getting married or being on the street as well. I had to think of my baby, so agreed to marry him, in order to have a roof over my head while I was pregnant.

I tried to leave him, but he treated me very abusive, in ways that I can't even begin to explain. I tried several time to leave him. My life got so bad that even all the cutlery and glassware plus all the extras that my Dad gave me, he sold. Every day I returned home from work something was not there anymore. Even my daughters' bed. I was so furious, but was too scared to act; he might just start hitting me again.

His physical abuse was done in the oddest ways. He would always start pushing me around first then start punching me in areas that won't show much bruising and was luckily easy for me to cover up with, without over dressing so that no one would notice.

After the last try, my husband sexually abused me and told me I deserve it. I went to the police and filed a complaint, but nothing came of it. A couple of months passed when I found out I were pregnant again. Then the abuse got worse, where I eventually believed everything was my fault.

I had two weeks to go before my due date and just experienced one of his session at home, I started to bleed, but luckily went away not long after. The next day he took me to go see my mother as he said that this would be the last time I will be allowed to see her. I went to the toilet, when I got up to flush the toilet it was full of blood. My mom phoned the hospital and they insisted that I come in. I did not say anything about the previous day's fight. It would be easier just to prevent another fight.

After my son was born, I tried once more to leave him, but did not succeed. When my son was only six months old I tried to leave him again. This time I succeeded with a little help from the police. I loved my children very much, and did not blame them for my life going wrong. It was just one of the many mistakes I have made in my life.

CHAPTER 2

Sarah making a new life for herself

I managed to survive the trauma that I experienced with soon to be ex-husband. I went to court to file for a divorce. When the day arrived that the divorce was going to be finalized, he never even pitched to fight for the kids. I was so happy when the divorce case was finalized, but also very disappointed for my children sake. I phoned him to ask him why he did not come to the court and why he did not fight for any rights on the kids. His words were "they are not mine, I don't want them". My heart was broken into pieces for the sake of my children. "Perhaps it was for the best, I really did not want my children to associate with a man like him". Not long after this I found out that he had passed away. I decided to start a clean slate with my children.

I left my last job for a fresh start, when I received a phone call to go for an interview at an international company. I dressed into my best clothes and left for the interview on a good note. The best attitude will bring the best results, I always believed.

I wore a green dress that complemented my skin. When I walked into the office, everybody had their heads turned my way, their eyes followed me as I walked though to the other side of the office where I glanced back and smiled. Tim fell in love with me at that moment. He has been divorced for six year at that time and never did a woman draw his attention like I did.

I was sitting at home so nervous of what to expect of the interview. I knew that I had to have the job otherwise I would have to ask for help from my Mother, this I did not want. This time I wanted to do things on my own, with no help. About two weeks later the call came though that I was waiting for. I got the job! I was so happy; Life can't get any better than this.

I had only two weeks left at home, before I started with my new job. That Monday morning I woke up, ecstatic to start my new job. I stood in front of my wardrobe, with tears in my eyes, there's not much in the wardrobe, but I made the best of what I had. I arrived at my new job, where everybody was helping me to get through my first day at work. I went home with such a good feeling about this company.

The next couple of weeks were all about learning about my job, as I did not have any experience in this line of work. I am very devoted and determined to make a success in my career, which I did everything in her power to learn what I could in a short time.

Months have passed, where I achieved more than I ever achieved in any of my employment. The company trusted me so much at this time, as the letters from my clients expressed how they enjoy working with me. My company was so impressed with my accomplishments they decided to send me on courses to advance my experience even more.

Jerry worked in the same department as me, he notice how I withdrawn I am from interacting too much with the staff. He sat me down, telling me that life is short, and I should enjoy every moment of it. He suggested that I should get out and date again. I am scared, because of what happened to me, so I ignored the comment and continued with my work.

Tim tried several times to invite me to join him outside for a smoke, but I preferred to smoke alone. Tim gave up and eventually followed me outside the one day to join me for a smoke; I smiled at him, but did not talk. This carried on for almost a week, when I opened up to Tim.

I was in the dark of how Tim felt about me. He always gazed at me, when I was working at my desk. The way he looked at me, it was like incredible—standing on a hill overlooking the ocean at sunrise, this was the way he saw my beauty. It is unexplainable, but amazing.

We had a lot in common and both went through a battered divorce, which we do not have much to show for. Tim was living with his Mom—Libby in rich town called Umhlanga Rock, not far from work. Wanda, his older sister lent her spare vehicle to him to get from work and back every day. It did not disturb Tim, not to have anything; he trusted in God that the next day would be provided.

Every day I woke up, feeling more and more secure about myself. It has taken a lot for me to build up my self-esteem again. Once you fall of a horse, it is hard to get back on the horse, but if you don't, you never will. I will always have that fear of trusting a man again.

I don't have a car license and also don't own my own car, and lived far away from work, I had to always arrange with someone in the office to take me home or even close to home, where I can call someone close by to fetch me. I managed to keep Amy and Ryan safe until I got home to feed and bath them. I always ensured that I spent at least an hour everyday with them, before they went to bed. With me staying by myself, I did not take well care of myself. I only worried about feeding my children. I never ate at home. My mother packed me a small lunch for work every day. That was all I ever ate and was getting skinnier by the day.

I was laying in bed the one night thinking of what Jerry said to me. "Perhaps he is right", I thought! It tends to get lonely at night once my kids have gone to bed. I have no one to talk to, only watch television. The following day I asked Tim if he could give me a lift home, he agreed. We enjoyed each other's company so much. I always tried to look happier than what I was. Tim asked me if he can do this one thing for me, to take some worries of my shoulders, as he saw it worried me every day. I accepted for Tim to take me home every day and pick my children up at the same time. I was so happy about this I actually was relieved.

The more we spent together, the fonder we grew of each other. Tim was taking me home for about two weeks now, when I invited him up for coffee. While I was preparing dinner for the children, Tim was entertaining the children in the bath. Once dinner was prepared I dried them and dressed them for dinner. I put down a plastic carpet mat for the kids so that could eat. In the meantime I ordered a pizza for Tim and myself. I felt that it is too late for Tim to go home and still eat. The kids went to bed not long after they ate.

We spent the rest of the evening getting to know each other. We spoke of everything in our lives, the bad and the good. The evening went very well, that we forgot about time for that moment and Tim ended up only going home close to midnight. Tim went straight to bed as he was tired and could not wait to go to work the next day.

I found out some days later that he was borrowing money from Sandy, his younger sister, so he can take me home. I was furious with him and confronted him. "Why did you not tell me that you can't afford it, I am surely someone that can understand this", Tim answered back "Sandy does not mind, she actually offered", but I was still upset with the whole idea of this. I felt that he should have told him.

I withdrew myself from Tim, and tried to prevent talking to him. Eventually Tim came up to me and said that I am acting childishly and should grow up. This upset Tim, as to how I was acting, but Tim did not understand why I was like this. I invited Tim for a smoke to explain to him how scared I am, that I might make the same mistake as I did it the past. "Tim I will rather walk away now, before I get hurt".

Their company had a farewell that Friday night, but I could not make it, as I had no one to look after my children. I was very disappointed not to be able to stay. Tim was heartbroken for days as I broke the friendship between us. Ravine gave Tim a couple of drinks to build up his courage to phone me and invite himself over for coffee, I did not accept. But I thought this was so sweet for him to phone me.

After a week of smiles and giggles, I decided to give it one more tries. It felt good that someone could make me feel this great. We got closer and closer over the weeks and spent more time together over the weekends too. Tim phoned me that Saturday morning to get ready; he was taking me with to the shops so he could introduce me to his family and his son—James. I am quite short and could not carry Ryan around the shops for a long time, as he was too heavy, he was also too small to walk by himself for a long time. Tim insisted that he carry Ryan. Tim's mother Libby was spending time with Amy and Ryan. James was a naughty little boy but in an adorable way.

We enjoyed the scenery and had lunch there. Libby always asked how the kids were after that day. She took a liking in Ryan. He had a personality that was very likable. We spent the whole day at the shopping mall, dropped me off afterwards. Tim walked me to the lift and said our good buys. About an hour later, my phone rang it was Tim. "Could you please open the door?" I ran to the door to open it, gave Tim a huge hug. The kid's were still awake and was excited to see him. They enjoyed Tim's' company.

I went to work after the weekend, with a great idea. I was standing outside waiting for Tim, to tell him what I wanted to do. I said to Tim, that I managed to get a babysitter and only this one time for that Saturday night. I wanted us to go out on a date, seem that we have been seeing each other for a while now, but have not been on a date.

Tim thought it was also a good idea; he was just as excited as I was. The week went slow—at last it is Friday. Tim notified Libby that he would be at my place for the night, as it is a bit far to travel too late at night, besides it is dangerous as well. Tim did not know my town at all, so he suggested that I make the choice as to where we should go.

Tim wants to go eat out, but I had other ideas. I took Tim to the local restaurant in town; we were both all of a sudden nervous. Strange how people get nervous when they realize that they know each other well enough to be comfortable, and when something like this happens they get nervous. I was too nervous to eat, so we ordered a couple of drinks. We left there and I decided to take him to a couple of Bars to show him the town. I was not use to drinking, as I have not had a drink in a long time and ended up getting very drunk.

Tim took me home, I stumbled out the car. Couldn't find my flat keys in my bag to unlock the gate and enter the building. Eventually I managed to get them; Tim took me up to my flat. The babysitter was asleep next to the kids on the bed. She woke up because of all the commotion in the flat. Luckily she was a friend of mine and said it was too late for her to go home, that she will spend the night.

I was standing in the passage, was swaying so much I fell back and bumped my head against the cupboard. Tim helped me back up and laid me down on my bed. The next morning I woke up with such a bad headache, I woke Tim up and apologized for my behavior. Tim did not tell me that he had an exam that morning, he had to rush out with such a speed otherwise he would have missed the class. I took the rest of the morning very easy, luckily Amy and Ryan was keeping themselves busy with their toys.

Tim phone me after his exam, we spoke for about an hour on the phone. I was so happy, that Tim was not upset about the night before. I knew that I embarrassed myself, and felt ashamed every time I thought of that time.

Chapter 3

Sarah moving in with Tim

Tim invited me to spend a weekend at his mom's place. I was nervous about the idea, but accepted the invitation. When it was Friday Tim took me home to pick my kids up and a few things from home. His mom insisted that I also bring my washing so that I can have it washed. It was so kind of her, as I did not have a washing machine. I washed the kids' clothes eve night when they went to bed. When I got there everybody was waiting in the driveway for us. I got out the car and Libby gave me a big hug, I smiled and carried on walking. Libby was talking to me while we were walking into the house and whispered to me "thank you for making her son so happy". She explained how he was always so miserable until he met me.

I was pleased that It made her happy. We spent the Friday night watching movies until late. Ryan was still in nappies and drinking from the bottle, so I had to get up during the night to change him and give him a fresh bottle of tea. Ryan loved his tea. When I was about to get up, Tim told me to get back in bed, he will sort Ryan out for me. It made me feel uncomfortable. Libby explained to me in the morning why Tim is like this. He is use to getting up for babies and found it odd for me to get up, as he was always the one to get up for James when Tim was still married to his ex-wife.

That following morning, Sandy and I sat around the pool while the kids were playing in the garden. Tim was on the other side of the house doing what he loved best, gardening. Tim took the kids for ice cream when he had finished with the garden. We all talked, laughed and enjoyed the rest of the day. Sunday morning Libby and everyone went to church. I decided to stay home as I had something I wanted to do, to surprise Libby. To thank her for a wonderful weekend. I cleaned up her house for her, and made the family a wonderful lunch. When they got home everything was done, all they had to do was sit down at the dining room table and enjoy their meal. It has been a while since I had so much fun.

After lunch Tim took us home. When Tim left and I walked into my flat I all of a sudden felt lonely. I missed being around Tim and his family. Amy and Ryan were tired of the weekend and just wanted to sleep. I put them to bed for a nap, woke them up after an hour. While running their bath water Amy asked me where Tim is. I explained to her that he has gone home. She said to me—"Why can he not live with us?" I tried to ignore the subject, as I did not want to get to use to Tim, as I was not sure where our relationship was headed.

Tim and his family enjoyed have us so much that we went there every weekend. This went on for two months, when Libby eventually phoned me to ask us to move in with them. She has gotten so use to the kids, whom she could not bear one more day without them and she enjoyed my company. I said yes, but did not tell her when I will be moving in. Tim arrived at my place the next night to fetch me. I had nothing packed, nothing ready to take.

One of my friends was visiting with a 4x4 so I asked her if she would mind helping me move. We had everything packed and ready to take down within an hour. Shows you, I did not have much. It was already dark and the kids were tired. When we got there Amy and Ryan's beds were already made for them so they could go to bed, while we were offloading and saying our good-byes.

Tim and I took everything inside. Tim showed me where I can put all my stuff. He already made space in his cupboard for me. It was so sweet of him.

The weekend after I moved in Amy and Ryan decided to have an art competition on the wall with black shoe polish. The room looked very creative. It took us two days to clean the walls and tiles on the floor. I was disappointed in my kids and did not know what to do. I sat in my room when Libby came in and said they are only kids, so don't punish them. Just have a good talk to them. We all in turn put away all the things that the kids could get hold off, this we did not want to experience again.

We were notified that her lease is up and has to move out of the house. Libby found a nice 4-bedroom house with a pool not far from this one. Amy got her own room and Ryan shared the main room with Libby as he was still small and it was the biggest rooms of all.

Sandy's twin brother Brad was coming down for a month, as it was their birthday. She had her own hairdressing business and was well off financially. Between the two of them they arranged for a big party at the house and invited everybody they knew. I helped Sandy choose a nice outfit for the party; she had someone in mind that she wanted to impress. That did not go so well when he decided not to pitch. The barbecue was busy going, drinks with a lot of snacks that was put out on the table until the barbecue was done.

We all danced, drank and had a lot of fun. When we woke up the next morning, the place was a mess. We were all suffering with a hangover and had to still clean the place up. Libby was nice enough to tell us to go lay down, she will clean up and look after the kids. We slept the day away; Libby woke us up about 15h00 with a big greasy meal to make us feel better. It worked, but when the night came we could not sleep, we slept too much.

Libby went to the shops every Saturday to buy food and stuff for the house. Guaranteed, she always came out the shop with something for the kids. The year was almost finished and had to find a pre-school for Amy. We decided to keep Ryan at home for another year as he was still too young to send and I could not afford it.

Amy made friends easily and fit in well at the school. She was invited often to birthday parties, but could not go to all of them, because it was difficult to explain every time to Ryan why he could not go. Libby helped me during the week to potty train Ryan, which helped me a lot. One less thing to worry about.

Sandy and I went to the pet shop to look at the cute kittens that just came in, Sandy had a love for cats, and she always walked out with one. This time I came out with a little ginger kitten, he was so adorable. The kitten did not live long, as he decided to go strolling that night and got hit by a car. Cats are very clever. One of our other cats brought him back, it took him three days. We took him to the vet, but did not make it. I promised myself that I would never have another cat; it broke my heart too much.

CHAPTER 4

Sarah gets married and fall ill for the first time

We have been living together just over a year now. It is Christmas morning; two hours until we leave for Church, the kids were as excited as this was their first real Christmas. Tim then decided that we must all open our presents first before we leave. I found it a bit suspicious, but went along with it. Once everybody opened their presents there was one small present left under the tree. I thought it was one of the ornaments from the tree, which had fallen off. So I took no notice. Tim picked it up and handed it over to me, he looked really nervous, "Is this mine?" I said, while opening it. I had already received so many gifts, I did not expect any more.

Tim leaned over and whispered in my ear "Will you marry me?" I was shocked. Everybody was waiting to see my reaction, as they all knew about it. They kept the secret very well. It took me a few seconds to get back to reality; I jumped up and wrapped my arms around Tim to give him a big romantic kiss. The kids were estranged with the whole situation, as they were too young to understand. We was so happy, Libby couldn't wait to tell everyone at Church. I wondered who was the more excited, them or me. When church finished, we had all the people around us, congratulating us

Libby decided that we should go out for lunch to celebrate our engagement, instead of eating a cooked meal at home like we always do. The kids loved this idea as they had a play area at the restaurant to keep them entertained. The moment was perfect, Amy and Ryan were enjoying themselves and so was everyone else.

I have never dated anyone that my family even remotely approved off. My family just loves Tim. Yes, he is a wonderful person and has a heart of gold. He would do anything for me. Our love was so great; we could not bear being one moment without one another. I would never expect myself to date or even marry someone like Tim. I always went to the wrong kind of men. This time I definitely made the right choice.

When Christmas was over and we got back to work, Tim and I told everyone at work that we got engaged. But sat with a predicament, one of us had to find a new job in a different company and two people are not allowed to be married and working in the same company. We were not too worried about this as we loved each other so much and besides we did not even set a date yet.

A couple of months have passed, when I fell ill for the first time since my school days. Tim took me to the doctor, and could find anything wrong with me and sent me home with anti-inflammatory tablets—little pink ones, which did nothing to me. I slept the whole weekend away, with not being able to spend time with my children nor Tim. I really felt bad about this, as I everyday make a point to spend at least a couple of hours with my family. I thought, "perhaps I am just having an off couple of days". I went back to work that Monday and told no one that I was very ill the weekend. Tim is the best thing that ever happened to me, besides my children. I have always had very healthy life; it was strange for me to have felt this way.

Sandy had a special surprise for me and arranged with Tim to drop me off at her work that Saturday morning. She booked a queens-day treatment for me at her hair and beauty salon, which she owned. I walked in, tea and cake was served. I had my hair washed, cut, colored and blow-dried. Afterwards the beautician, who she gave me a bikini, leg and underarm wax, took me. From there I was taken to be seated to have a manicure and a pedicure. I understand now why they call it the queens-day, because you go home feeling like one.

I was fine for a couple of months when I fell ill again. This time I felt worse than the last time, I was so week that I could barely walk. Tim was really worried about me this time and took me back to my doctor to see if he would do any tests to find out why I am getting like this, but he insisted that I don't need any tests. He then gave me this big speech, making it sound so real and making us believe it telling me there is nothing wrong with me, so he sent me back home, again with the pink tablets and was booked of sick for a week. He thought that I was just exhausted and needed extra rest. All I did was sleeping that week; I could not even get out of bed to go to the toilet and hardly ate. So this made me even weaker. I eventually recovered, from I don't know what, and went to work.

My career was going very well; to be honest I think I was at my peak of my career. I really knew my work, not even my manager could catch me out. They even decided to add more to my work load with extra responsibilities. He even trusted me with some financial responsibilities, but obviously my salary did not get increased. I believed that I will get what I deserve in due time. It was hard to accept all this without an increase, I even thought of leaving the company several times. But nothing came of it. I enjoyed by job too much and knew that there was more to learn, so I remained with them.

It was time for Ryan to go to school as well. He was the type of person that everybody just had to like him. Ryan came home the one day talking about his Dad. I got a bit nervous and asked him "your dad, who is this now"; he commented back "Uncle Tim is my Dad". Since that day Ryan always called Tim, Dad. Ryan from a small age called Libby his Nanna, which made her very happy as it means granny from where she came from. Libby was born and raised in England.

Tim decided to get me interested in some hobbies to entertain my mind. Sandy showed me some ornaments that she painted a long time ago and asked me if I would be interested in doing this. I thought it would be nice, something completely different to doing nothing. Tim took Sandy and me to go buy some ornament and paint so we could go painting when we got home. Sandy still had some paint left from the previous once she painted. We only had to buy a few extra colors. I enjoyed it so much, I was painting every chance I could get, and Sandy enjoyed it as well. She originally stopped because she had no one to paint with. This brought us even closer which was a good thing.

I painted so many ornaments; Tim displayed them on a rack where everybody could see them. He was so proud of what I have done. Every Sunday after Church, we would go to the flea market down the road from us, to go buy ornaments and paint, which was so much cheaper that buying in an art shop. Amy and Ryan loved this as they had a playground where all the children would play while their Moms and Dads were walking around the stalls. They even had a live band and food stalls, so you could spend the whole day there.

One Sunday after we got home from the flea market, Tim's' ex-family was waiting there. We invited them in for tea and coffee, we enjoyed their company so much that we insisted that they stay for dinner. Tim loved when they came over, as James was living with them, and did not see much of him. He enjoyed every minute they could together. As we did not have much money, Tim could rarely go visit James. They came to visit often after that day. They would come on a Friday night and spend the whole weekend. We enjoyed their company as they appreciated life as it was given to them.

A week after they came to visit, I fell ill again with constant headaches. The doctor prescribed pain tables and sent me home. The headaches wouldn't go away, so I went back. He could find nothing wrong with me physically and carried on as if I was imagining it. I was very angry when I left there, but looked at Tim and it reminded me of what a great life I have. I tried to live with the headaches, but some days were harder than other days.

CHAPTER 5

Moving into their own place

Our lease was up and had to move as the owner wanted to sell the house and needed to do some renovations to the place before he could do sell. Libby had some contacts at the rental agency, so she managed to get a good deal with a 6 bedroom double storey house literally down the road. It was perfect; there were 2 bedrooms and a bathroom down stairs, three bedrooms, a double study room and two bathrooms upstairs. Ryan eventually had his own room after all this time.

It eventually came to the day that we had to move. Sandy managed to get a couple of guys to help us move. Even though we had a lot of stuff to move, it was pointless to hire a truck as it was just down the road.

Only after we moved into this house did we realize all the problems the place had, but we made them best of it. We also learned that one of the guys that were helping us move was seeing Sandy secretly. He eventually admitted it and started coming around more often. They would sit in the lounge till late at night talking.

Ryan slept in the one and we slept in the other room down stairs. Amy, Sandy and Libby slept upstairs. The house had a small garden so Tim did not have much to maintain. The pool was smaller and shallower that the one in the previous house so it was safer for the children to swim in. They still could not swim properly. Someone always had to be there, before they were allowed to swim. I enjoyed swimming and often joined them in the pool.

I have now developed a bump on my head; it was not that big, but big enough to get worried about, and still with my headaches continuing I started getting very concerned about it. Tim took me to the doctor straight away when I made him feel the bump. The doctor felt the bump asked me if I bumped my head, but I did not. He said it is a deformation of my head. I walked out and said to Time, "I would have known if it has been there long". I started thinking, "Perhaps it is my imagination". One thing I do know is that the headaches is real and then realized that the doctor did not even say anything about my headaches.

Sandy owned two dogs Blue & Sky; they were always locked up in the back as we always had guests over and were not too fond of new people. They were not allowed in the front garden and started to get very aggressive due to one of them being female and were on heat. The only time they were calm is when there was more than one adult around. Tim was busy doing some gardening and the children were playing in the garden where he was. Amy decided to tease blue, he got tired of it, when Amy went again to touch him he turned around and bit her under her arm. We cleaned it very well with some Dettol. Luckily it did not look to serious, but still took Amy to the doctor in the morning to have it looked at and so that she could get a Tetanus injection. I am sure Amy learnt her lesson not to tease dogs.

Not long after I have been to the doctor I fell ill again, now the doctor is saying I suffer from migraine ore's. I could not believe what I was hearing. The way he was explaining how it works sounded so real and believable. I was so tired of getting ill so often, I sometimes thought I was going mad and imagining things.

Tim and I decided that it was time to move into our own place. We first decided to start getting the most important things that we need to start with for our place, like kitchenware, bedding and the odd thing. We also received a couple of things for our wedding which helped a lot. We felt that we did not need too much, that we would get most of it once we have a place.

We eventually found a place in my hometown, as we could not afford living by ourselves and sending the kids to school in the area Libby was living—it was too expensive. It was a far travel everyday to work, but cost wise it was so much cheaper to live there. The flat that we found was perfect for us. It had three bedrooms, two bathrooms and a double garage, and it was cheap for size of the flat. The view was to die for, with a full 180degrees view of the ocean.

We moved in over a weekend, as we did not have much to take over. Tim and I went the day before to go buy a fridge and arranged for it to be delivered that same day we arrive at the flat. Libby lent us two sleeping couches so we had something to sleep on. My mother lent us two chairs so we would have something to sit on into the lounge. We have never been this happy in our lives. Even though we had nothing, we had everything that was needed to survive. Amy had a bed to sleep one; Ryan had a sleeper couch in his room just like us. The most important thing was we were happy. We had our own place!

We could basically do what we wanted, not always worry about what the others are doing. Libby eventually moved out of the big house into a small Granny flat, that she and Sandy shared. By now Sandy and Charles have gotten engaged and making plans for the big day. I was very happy for them. I always thought it was about time. Sandy did not date anyone from the time Tim and I started seeing each other. I know she liked a guy that worked nearby her shop, but he broke her heart.

The kids often went to visit Libby there as they missed her so much. They were so use to have their Nanna around them, spoiling them with treats and gifts. Amy used to wake up early in the morning and played in her room till everyone was up. Since we have been in our own place she has been sleeping later and later. It pleased me very much, as it concerned me that she was not getting enough sleep.

Ryan was still struggling to sleep on his own, as he was use to sharing a room with Libby. When we moved into our flat, we only learned that he would sneak out at night and sleep with his Nanna. Early hours of the morning she would wake him up and put him back in his own bed. As of this result we struggled with this for a couple of months and eventually got him to sleep in his own bed the whole night. The night-light helped dramatically for him to get use to sleeping by himself. Every night he slept by himself we would reward him.

The only thing that had me worried was being on the ninth floor with two small children. Their bedrooms also had sliding doors to their balconies. So I locked it and forbid them to go out without adult supervision. Luckily they obeyed this one big rule I gave them. They were still small but had to be told from the day we moved in that the going outside in not allowed.

The flat started to get furnished slowly but surely. As Tim and I could no long handle sleeping on the sleeper couch? Tim often woke up with a sore back and my body was always aching because of it. So we went and bought a second hand bed from a guy at work. My mom bought us a second hand lounge suite so the kids did not have to sit on the floor anymore. It took us just over a year to get our place furnished. It wasn't perfect furnisher but it did the job that's all that mattered.

The bump on my head was getting bigger so I decided to get a second opinion. I did not have a good medical aid and would only cover the doctors where my doctor is. So I made an appointment to see a different doctor. He had a look at the bump and was a bit concerned. He had some blood test taken, but nothing showed in the blood. He was not willing to go further with this either, but suggested I have a look at it.

CHAPTER 6

Sarah always being sick

I decided to go to my old family doctor, to see what he would suggest as nobody wants to help me find out what is wrong with me. He had blood taken and showed that my white blood cells are down so he suggested that I probably busy getting flu or something. He did not mention anything about the bump on my head. It was frustrating that no one wants to do something about the bump on my head, nor the headaches. He is pretty old so I thought; I'll forgive him this time. By know I have been suffering with headaches for a year and a half, 24/7. Life at home for Tim has become very stressful as he could not help me feel better. Tim was one of those people who would make a serious thing look funny. He was always joking to try and make things look better than what they are. Tim and I are the two happiest people in the world, regardless of me always feeling ill.

Tim and I carried on with our lives as if nothing was wrong, to prevent the kids from noticing that something is wrong. But not knowing, they already notice and asked Tim "Why does Mommy get sick so often?" We always changed the subject to happy thoughts so that we did not have to discuss this topic, not even we knew why. I love my children very much and always try to protect them things like this that not even I understand.

The only way I would forget about me always getting sick is to pretend that I am feeling fine and not always sick, as I feared that I might lose everything good in my life just because I am sickly. So I got up one morning early, sat on the balcony with a cup of tea and enjoyed the early sunrise. I sat there until the sun was aligned with the sea. It was the most beautiful sight. It looked like a silver road to the sun. I woke Tim up with a cup of coffee and gave him a big kiss. Went to the kitchen and made my family a big breakfast, not something I usually do on Sunday.

During the week was better for me as my workload kept my mind casted on my work and not letting my mind wonder. I believed that I was fine and that everything is fine. Then only did I start living again. Tim and I dropped off Amy and Ryan at my Mom's for the night, while we went to dinner with a view overlooking the ocean. The moon casted over the sea. It was very peaceful with just the sound of the wave braking on the shore. We enjoyed each other's company so much, like nothing before. The next morning we were both up early to enjoy the sunrise. This was not one of the main reasons why we were up early; it was that we are so use to having the kids around that it felt strange and lonely.

Everything was going well until I had a black out on the steps at work. This caused for me to lose my balance and fall. Luckily I did not get hurt seriously. This was when the 5 second black out session started. I was still aware of what was going on, I just couldn't see through my eyes. It was similar to a dark evening when someone decides to switch the light off for a few seconds. At first I did not take much notice of it, because I thought it was only dizzy spells as everybody gets them know and again.

Work was very concerned and sent me home and insisted that I find out what caused me to collapse. I went to my family doctor again.

He examined my body, had a look at the bump on my head, which was getting bigger by the day and had more blood test, done. He sent me home and insisted that I come see him a week later.

It was the most unpleasant feeling. I kept quiet for a long time until I could no longer handle it. It started happening more often and for lengthy times. While I would walk I had to grab hold of the closest object so that I can stand still until it went away. I eventually told Tim what was going on, he was so angry with me for not telling him. We kept a close eye on how frequent I would get them. I tried to ignore the situation as much as possible.

The week went well with no incidents of feeling ill or collapsing. I went back that Friday to get my blood results, he was not happy. My white blood cells were lower that the last blood test. He gave me a letter and said I can have the bump removed locally as soon as possible, he said it was not harmful so I don't have to worry but it needs to be removed. I suggested that this was the cause of me feeling ill and why my white cells were so low. I explained that my medical aid would not accept for me to go to any hospital, so he wrote a letter to the hospital that my medical aid covered.

I did not worry about the bump, and any signs of feeling ill as the doctor said it was not serious. The only distraction was my black outs that I got. After a while it did not disturb me anymore and said to Tim, that I will see how things go before I go for this local removal of the bump.

I carried on like this for a further six month, when I collapse in the shower. My kids misunderstood the commotion and thought that Tim caused for me to get hurt in the shower. Amy went to school and told everybody that her Dad broke her mommy's arm. This caused so much havoc at school, Tim was called in and had to explain what happened. We spoke to Amy and explained that I collapsed in the shower and her

Dad had nothing to do with it, he was not even there when it happened. I had to comfort her and make her understand that her Dad loves me very much. Ryan was luckily a bit too young to understand what was going on, but had him involved in the conversation so he would understand.

My bump was quite big now, headaches were getting worse and so was my black outs. I went to search on the website with all my symptoms and came up with so many things that could be wrong. I should not have done this as it caused me to be very concerned and made me worry so much that I got very sick.

Tim insisted that I go to the hospital to have this sorted before it gets so bad that I lose my job. I then had no choice, as I did not want my kids to suffer financially because of my stubbornness. I asked Tim if we could go in months' time as my workload we very busy and cannot afford to take off work at the moment.

CHAPTER 7

She finally gets some results

We arrived at the hospital, inquired in reception where we should go and arrange for this to be done. Even though my doctor said that this should be a local surgery no one knew what I was talking about. The lady insisted that I see a nero specialist because it was on my head. He insisted that go and have a CT Scan done to the area where the bump is.

My medical aid did not cover to have this done at this hospital unless I am booked in. I went to a government hospital, but still had to pay out of my pocket to have the CT scan done. After waiting for 4 hours I eventually had this done and went back to see the nero specialist. He was already closed and his receptionist insisted I come back the next day.

I was there bright and early that following morning with my scan. He had a look at is and refused to do surgery on the bump. He said it is a lump and has pushed down but the scan could not show how far down and if it was attached to my brain. The doctor referred me to a neurosurgeon to have a look at it. By know I was feeling so depressed as I have been pushed from one side to another and can't get any straight answers from anybody.

Tim and I sat outside the hospital feeling hopeless; as it is our medical aid will not cover the doctor at that hospital nor will they cover any operation at this hospital. We were out of options and did not know what to do. Do we go ahead and pay out of our own pocket or do we go home. We could not afford to pay out of our own pocket as we were barely making it through financially every month.

We took a chance, and made the appointment to go see the neurosurgeon. When we arrived there it was very understanding. He had a look at the CT scan, and insisted on having a MRI done. I once again had to explain my medical aid problem, that they only cover certain doctors and hospitals. He assured me that I need not to worry about this.

He did some physical tests and the sent me for a MRI to see how far and big this lump is, because the CT scan did not show it properly. I had to sit and wait in his rooms till the results came back. While all this was done his secretary was on the phone with the medical aid to see what our options were. She did not get many results from them, but kept on trying. The doctor called me back in with the MRI results. He was not happy at all.

The lump has pushed though my scull and attached itself to my brain. He needed to have it removed ASAP. He also did a physical examination to see what effects this tumor has on me. He then insisted that I have it removed straight away. The medical aid was being very difficult, at first they refused for me to be booked into this hospital, but his receptionist fought with them and explained if I do not have this operation it will end up being life threatening.

At this stage I was so scared that I blocked out anything that was going on around me and tried to think of happy things. The medical aid eventually after an hour of fighting gave the doctor 3 days to do the entire test that is necessary and then they will pay for the operation.

They pushed two weeks of tests into three days, to see if there were any other growths or anything else wrong. I felt like a lab rat literally. I was poked with needles, had every scan that you can think of and still have not seen the doctor after a full day. The nurse came to me and explained that I will be going into Theatre the following morning. I was a bit concerned as no one said anything about the medical aid as it has been three days and still has not had the surgery.

Tim came to see me at the hospital everyday. I was missing my kids so much and wanted them to come and see me, but Tim felt that it would do them more harm than good, he was right. He was struggling to cope as he was so use to me doing everything at home. My Mom decided to take Ryan for a couple of days to make things easier for him at home. My Mom would pick both the kids up from aftercare, bath them and feed them. So when Tim comes back from the hospital, all he had to do was give Amy something to drink before bed and send her to bed.

The day before the operation the doctor came to see me to explain the surgery and also explained all the consequences the operation could have. If I don't go for the operation I could land up in a Coma and if I do go for it, I could still land up in a Coma. It was a 50/50 chance. I could also land up like a vegetable, but had good faith that nothing will go wrong. He had to give me the breakdown as it was his job and that we needed to understand the dangers of the operation. He then drew circles around the tumor; he called it pre-pre-preparations. The nurses woke me up at 5h00 the next morning to go and have a shower and put this horrible smelling liquid in my hair. I was not allowed to rinse it; it had to stay in for the operation. I was told that I was not allowed to have a smoke but my nerves were finished and need to be calmed. I explained my predicament to the nurse and said that it will not be her responsibility; I am going out at my own risk.

I was not too bothered about her comments and still went for a smoke, while I was out smoking she phoned the doctor and explained her. He suggested that I lie down and relax in the bed. He also prescribed a tablet that calmed me. That was the last that I could remember before the operation.

After three hours of surgery, the lump was sent off for tests. I was sent to ICU afterwards, I cannot remember much from the time I was in ICU, but I know I was fighting wanting to go for a smoke when I woke up. Tim was there with me trying to explain I have a lot of pipes in my head and by my throat so there was nothing he could help me with. I was out for the rest of the day. I woke up the next morning feeling great, I just wanted my catheter out as I hated the feeling of it, putting pressure on my bladder. The nurse wiped me down and gave put some jelly and custard in front of me to eat. I was not allowed to leave unless I have eaten. I was starving so I ate it and asked for more.

They were so happy with my results and were released to the Nero ward that same day. Before I could leave a guy came and took some blood and gave me an Aids talk. I was still confused at that stage and did not bother me what he was talking about. I needed a toilet when I got there, but was still weak so they put a bedpan under me so I could relieve myself. When the curtains got opened up my Mom was waiting with some clean clothes and toiletries to go for a bath. I got out of bed, but struggled to walk as my body was very weak from surgery. My Mom bathed me and helps me get dressed. She did not have much time as she had to go back to work. She helped me back to my bed and left.

It was such a relief that the pain in my head had gone. The operation could not be compared with the pain that I suffered and eventually learned to live with it. I felt like a new person with so many possibilities in life.

Once my mother had gone, I wanted to go for a smoke, but the nurses felt that it was a bit too early for me to go out by myself and smoke. She insisted that I go later when I have accumulated some more energy. I was very determined so I went out for a smoke on my own risk, when I was finished smoking I felt unsteady. I definitely had to stay out here for a bit longer till I felt better. When I reached the reception area I fell down. The security guard helps me back up onto a wheel chair and pushed me back to my ward. The nurses were furious with me, they suggested that I start acting responsible and look after myself.

The ward started getting full and they needed my bed, so they transferred me to the same ward that I was in before the surgery. I preferred it there as it was not so open and only had three beds in. I looked at myself in the mirror and noticed that half of my hair was shaved away. I could not sleep either because of the rubber elastics they had put in my hair, it was hurting my head. I insisted that someone must cut the pigtails off. I was so relieved when they were out. I looked terrible, but I felt better. I had this big white bandage on my head and could not wash my hair. It was dirty and full of blood.

The following morning the doctor came to see me, he said that the operation went very well, but could not remove everything as he was too scared to go to close to my brain. He tried to remove as much as he could. He clarified that I have Non Hopkins Lymphoma and is treatable with success. I did not know what it was, but everyone looked so positive about it that it did not feel like I needed to have any concern. He asked that I come and see him within two weeks from date of operation, in order that I can have the pins removed from my head. He will no longer be handling my case and handing me over to another doctor that is more qualified in this field. Furthermore she will be seeing me the following day.

The nurses did not clarify with me what it is; all they mentioned was that it is curable. Not one person wanted to sit down with me and clarify as to what it actually wrong. I felt once again frustrated with suspense to find out what is wrong. I spent the rest of the day up and down the corridor going for smokes.

The new doctor came early the next morning to see me. I was still confused with the whole situation; she too did not clarify what Non Hopkins Lymphoma was. I was fed up with this whole situation. She pushed for two more test out of the medical aid, but only managed to get one more done. Before she left she handed over her card to me in order for me to book an appointment with her rooms once I have booked out of the hospital.

CHAPTER 8

Diagnosed with Non Hopkins Lymphoma

Before Tim came to take me home from the hospital, with it being still early I asked him if he would take me to Sandy to have my hair under control, with the center of my head having very little hair Sandy managed to blend my hair in nicely. We finished our tea and left for home to see my kids, I was as excited as I have not seen them for a long time

Ryan was constantly asking why my head looks like train tracks, I burst out with laughter as he had a good point and it was with such a seriously face. I made it clear to both the children that I had a big operation and removed the bump on my head. It had to be put in the simplest terms for them to understand the seriousness on the operation that I undergone.

The company I work for invited me to their Christmas function, even though I was not at the time at work. Each one was very concerned about me. Tim was boasting about the tracks on my head, which was covered with a bandanna at that time to protect my scar from direct sunlight. I felt more comfortable for me not to display the pins and besides it was more appropriate especially in front of the top Directors that were down here for the function.

I went to have the pins removed from my head a few days before the day I was suppose to have come, which fell over a weekend. For every pin that was removed a tear rolled down my cheek from the pain. I tried not to show it, but by the time last one was about to be pulled out, I screamed with excruciating agony, I in turn apologized profusely. The doctor re-examined me and was quite pleased with him. I could not thank him enough for what he had done for me.

Two weeks later I made an appointment with the new doctor. On her card it mentioned cancer center, which in turn concerned me a bit as no one mentioned anything about cancer to me. I kept this thought to myself especially from Tim; I don't think he could handle anything like this. "Perhaps it is not cancer and that she practices at different rooms for different things".

The time came to go see her, my mother offered to take me as Tim was working and could not get away from work that day. She came in with me to in case I need to be comforted. There was only one question I had on my mind the whole time I was sitting in the waiting room. They called my name and went in. The minute I sat down I inquired straight away before she could even say anything, "Do I have cancer?" She replied and confirmed yes very calmly. She did insist that I go for the test I could not go for in the hospital—a bone marrow biopsy, she can't determine how far the cancer has spread if I did not have this done. It was the only way she will be able to determine what type of treatment and course is required to help fight the cancer off.

There were so many things going through my mind at that moment, which I did not even here a word she said. She arranged to see me again in two weeks time. We left for home there was complete silence in the car. I don't think my mom knew what to say to me in order for me to feel better. I knew that I had to phone Tim and was going over and over how to explain to Tim that I have cancer. I eventually managed to build up enough courage to phone him, I pick up my cell phone, hearing the ringing in my ear made my heart beat sound even louder. Tim answered; I started crying on the phone when I explained to him that I have cancer. There was silence on the other side of the phone. "Are you okay", I asked. Tim said to me that he has to go and made an excuse that he has something urgent that he had to sort out for the big boss.

I needed only his comfort to make me feel better. When Tim arrived home he gave me a big hug, now this is all I needed the whole day. Tim handles problems in a different way than most people. He sat me down and said we will beat this and did not mention Cancer, once after this. This was not the first time Tim has confronted someone with cancer, his father passed away with Lung Cancer. Deep down I know this brought back bad memory of the past. I did not push him to talk and left him to deal with it in his own way.

It was time for me to go for my bone marrow biopsy, but yet again my medical aid did not cover this biopsy. I had to pay cash to have it done which was a bit cheaper where she recommended—directly at the labs itself. We picked up Libby before we went to the lab, in order to help me when I get home with the kids. She was the best mother-in-law anyone could ask for.

I arrived there not knowing what to expect, as it is one thing that I never had done. They gave me a calming tablet half an hour before they did the biopsy, so that I would not shake while they were doing it. All I felt was a bit of pressure in my lower back, I was still very nervous but with a bit of help from Libby holding my hand and comforting me it all went very quick and smooth. I had to sit for 10 minutes before we could go home just in case I started bleeding again. They suggested that I lay flat down on my back to put some pressure on the wound.

After a while I fell asleep on the bed, when I woke up I was in so much pain I could not get out of bed. He slept on the floor as he was scared that if he moved that it would hurt me, and had to be nearby so that if I needed to go to the toilet that he was right there to help me. Libby stayed with us for a couple of days to help out with dinner and things around the house until I was up and walking again. This carried on for about three day when I eventually could walk again and carried on with my daily routine.

The doctors' rooms called that my results are back and that I need to be there next week Monday, seeing that she need some time to get the correct treatment method that would suit me ready before my appointment. She diagnosed me with Stage 4 Non Hopkins Lymphoma, the aggressive type. She explained that there is an 80% survival rate for this type of cancer and is easier to cure than a slow growing cancer. The cancer was in my bone marrow and some was left on my brain, which could not be removed that will also require treatment. She has planned for an 8-month cycle of chemotherapy following with Radiotherapy treatment.

Tim asked her how long I would be off work for, because we still need my salary. We will not be able to survive with just one salary. She suggested that I take a year of work and that I needed the extra few months to recover from the trauma that my body will be going through. When we left I mentioned to Tim that he needs to take me to work so that I can speak to my boss and see if I am going to lose my job. I needed to resolve this so that we can plan our lives.

Not long after I was diagnosed we asked Libby to move in with us as we did not know how I would be after my treatments and needed help with Amy and Ryan. She moved in with us after two weeks of asking her. This took a lot of pressure of me, especially when I am ill, that there is someone to cook for Tim and the kids.

CHAPTER 9

Preparing for Treatment (Chemo)

The company was kind enough to keep me employed, while on treatment for the 8 months and still pay my salary every month. I was so grateful and lucky to be supported at this time of difficulty in my life.

The doctor wanted me to go on a higher or different medical aid, as they don't cover this treatment on the one that I am on. So Tim decided that I cancel mine in order to go on his so that I can receive my treatment. Everything was still a blur for me and hard to accept but tried to carry on with my life as if nothing was wrong. I think with feeling so sick for such a long time, it prepared me for what was about to happen to me.

I was asked to be early for my first treatment so that they could get me prepared and explain how it is going to work. I arrived just before they opened up, very nervous not knowing what to expect as everything is new to me. One thing I did notice from the previous visit that they are very warm and caring people that work there.

Tim and I sat in reception waiting for the nurses to get everything set before going through, my stomach was turning, and hands were sweating. I took a deep breath, just calming down the nurse called me in. Walking down the passage, feeling like the walls closing in on me, not being able to see the end of the passage, I felt very small at the point in time. Eventually I arrived where the patients have their treatment. The coldness of the room hit me, giving me chills down my arms. I don't remember feeling this scared the last time I was here. As I took a seat I silently prayed for help through the treatment.

They had the most beautiful leather reclining chairs for the patients that spent their time there, there was also a separate room that was more private from the open room for more patients, and I think it is used for the ones who have not yet accepted they have cancer.

As I was the first there I managed to get the best chair there. The nurse took my blood and asked me to wait in order to see if my system is ready for treatment today. Luckily it was fine; I just wanted to get it over and done with. First she explained what all the drip feeds were for and what the tablets were before she continued. My medication I had to take first which was for pain and nausea. About 10 minutes afterward they brought the needles to have the drip feed set up; at first they could not find a vein to insert the needle. Feeling sleepy and cold, the nurse provided a blanket and offered something to drink. At the time all I wanted to do, is to be left alone so I could sleep. We did not know how long the treatment would like, so Tim stayed with me to give me some comfort.

I ended up after 8 sachets of treatment staying a full day. The trip home I was feeling very bloated and swollen from all the liquid pushed into my system. I didn't feel like talking to any one, not being around people. When I got home I went straight to my room, closed the door and slept the night away. Tim made me a cup of tea the next morning and let me be. The kids were a bit eager to see me, so I insisted that they will only calm down if they have seen me and said a few words. Tim allowed them in only for a few minutes.

I did not know how my day would turn out so I rather stayed in bet. This was nothing like on the movies that you see they constantly sick, so far I have been very lucky. The nausea tablet given I did not feel that I needed to take them either. On the third day after my treatment my aching body was so severe that no one could come near me, insisting them to stay away. Furthermore I dare not to eat anything since the sores in my mouth was impossible to bear. The aching body and mouth sores continued for several days when finally I could eat with actually appreciating the taste of food again.

I went to work for the first time since the operation and cancer, everyone was concerned for me. Trying to help me as much as they could. At first they wanted to send me home, but gave in when I explained why I need to be here. I could not bear being at home with my mind that keeps wondering off, besides have people around me, once I was over the pain and everything, it was some sort of comfort to me. I did not want to sit at home feeling sorry for myself, I needed to get out and be with people. My hair started falling out slowly after the first treatment. I was blessed to have my hair short so it was not that bad falling out.

My time was up being at work and get ready for my next treatment. I was not looking forward to it, but knew it had to be done. Back in the chair again trying to find a vein, the nurse suggested that I have a port put in. This I was not to keen on, as there was so many problems that you occur with the port. I did not even think twice about it. We started a bit late this time, as they were very full. Sleeping the whole day away again, feeling a bit worse this time. I put on a brave face pretending that I am fine. Tim could not stay this time and had to go to work.

The side effects were the same, but my hair on my head was getting thinner every time. I eventually started to wear a scarf around my head. I could not afford to buy a wig. Besides Tim always liked me being real and not pretend to be someone else. I liked this about Tim because it made me realize and appreciate the natural beauty of a person.

After the 5th treatment, I had no hair on my head or my body. The only place my hair did not fall out was my eyebrows. For this I was very grateful. The color of my skin was also still normal. I was very grateful for the hair falling out on my legs and under my arms as I did not have to shave for whole time I was on treatment and my side effects were small compared to most cancer patients. I was very fortunate in this regard.

CHAPTER 10

More treatment (Radiotherapy)

Finally the day has come for my last treatment of chemotherapy. I had a scheduled time to see my doctor, while having my treatment to discuss any problems or concerns. She was very happy with my progress, as she did not expect everything to have gone this well. She asked when I am finished with my treatment to make an appointment to see her in two weeks time.

I went home after making the appointment, feeling very happy and relieved. I decided to stay up that night instead of lying down like I usually do after my treatments. Spent some time with my family and showed my gratitude towards Libby for always being there when I needed her. My children stayed up a little later that usual since this was a very special day for all of us. I survived the chemotherapy.

I had to meet my doctor at the hospital instead of at her rooms in order to make a mask for the radiotherapy treatment that I will be undergoing. While we were there, she explained that the hospital is very full and will not get the proper treatment that I require. She suggested a medical center that has space for me and will arrange for me to have my treatment there.

They took me into a dark room where the moulds get made, looking very scary. I was asked to lay facing down. With me having a phobia for confined space, I explained it was not possible, especially if this mould pushing me down. My heart started pounding and body shaking, my doctor whispered "we need to do this and you need to be strong for me. You have come so far, just to turn back now". I tried everything in my power to stay as calm as possible. After this incident I was definitely not looking forward to my treatment.

I went to work for a couple of days to distract my mind from speculation. My manager George was so happy to see me as they were struggling so much without me. The next morning he asked me if I would come to the boardroom with him. George and Jerry prayed over me for the cancer to go. It made me feel so good, ready for life.

The dreadful day has arrived for me to go for my first radiotherapy treatment. The room was dark and very big, in the centre of the room was the bed that I had to lay on. My mask was lying on the one side ready. They asked me to lay face down, strapping the mask in. I started to panic, as I did not feel in control any more. She came back loosened it a bit and asked me that I really need to stay still. The longer it propone the treatment the longer it will take to complete. It was the longest five minutes of my life.

When I had finished I was asked if I would like to see a physiatrist, but insisted that I was fine. All I wanted to do was get out of there, as far away as possible. I was not certain in what way this treatment was going to affect me, therefore went home. This carried on everyday for two weeks, with no affects. I felt there was no reason for me to stay at home anymore and rather work.

It was the scariest time in my life to find out if I still have cancer or if the treatments actually worked. In order to confirm that it has all gone tests needed to be done. My doctor scheduled appointments for me to have these tests done and one more to see her after it all. My first appointment was for another bone marrow biopsy, this time was done in the hospital. Again Libby came to help comfort me by holding my hand,

The pain was unbearable this time as they struggled to get the equipment threw my bone to draw the marrow in order to send for tests. The following week I went for a MRI to ensure that the tumor has gone and not started again. I was tired of all this back and forth, I just wanted to live a normal life.

My doctor phoned me to arrange to go for some blood tests three days before my appointment with her. The big day has come to find out my results, I was very nervous that morning before I arrived at her rooms, but self-assured at the same time. I have not come this far in my life to have more bad news.

I sat in reception waiting patiently to go in. Only waiting for an hour eventually Tim and I went in. She looked over the results and said things are looking good, but first she would like to give me a physical exam. I went though and sat on the bed while she was still talking to Tim. She looked at my scar on my head and looked in all the areas where Lymphoma might re-appear. She found nothing and suggested I go sit down.

She complemented me on how brave I have been through all this, but such confidence. I was getting very anxious about my results but tried not to show it. After a long lengthy discussion eventually she came to the point that I was waiting for. My blood, MRI and bone marrow result was very positive and confirmed I am now in remission. I jumped up with joy, thanking her for everything she has done for me.

She reminded me that I must come for regular check-ups to ensure that my cancer does not come back, but if it does that we can catch it in time.

They don't explain to you how it will be afterwards. The best things you can do are embrace life with open arms and enjoy it. Try not to think of what you have been through, rather live for the future. You have a second chance in life so take it.

I am now in remission for the forth year and enjoying every moment of it with my family.

www.ingramcontent.com/pod-product-compliance
Lightning Source LLC
Chambersburg PA
CBHW050343290526
45785CB00006B/2607